Just Love 4 Tennis Kids

THIS BOOK BELONGS

TO: _____

By

Coach Rachelle Lifpitz

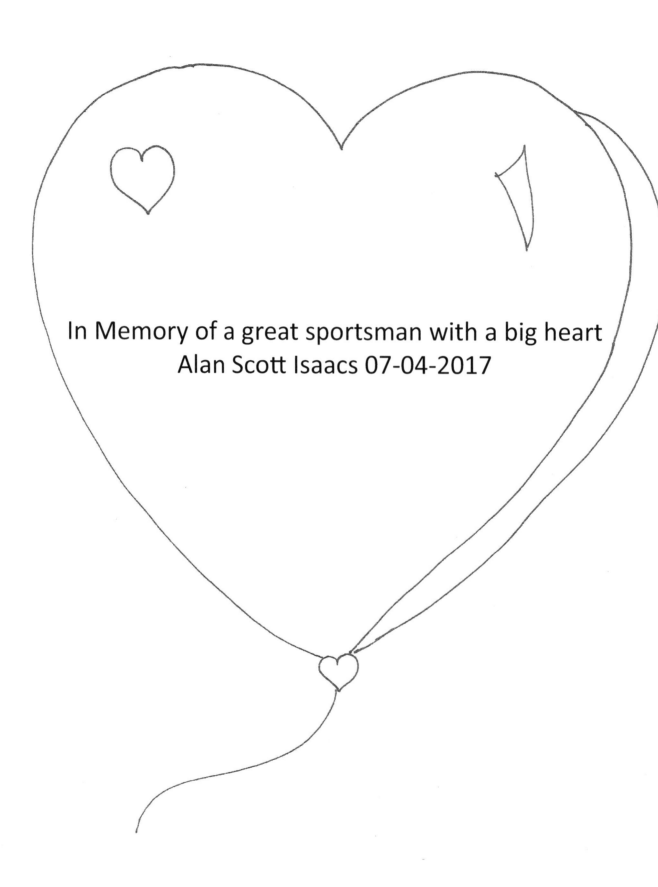

I wrote this tennis book in memory of my brother, Alan Scott Isaacs who passed away on July 4 2017.

We used to call Alan big A.I. because he was our big hero! May he rest in peace.

Alan loved all types of sports. He especially loved to play the game of tennis.

He was a salesman for Nike for many years and he was known as the guy that would "Just Do It!"

In his passing, he would have wanted all of us to "Just Love" the game of tennis because the whole idea of playing tennis to him was to play and have fun with friends and family.

The reason I wrote this book is to help families and friends learn to enjoy the game of tennis. Tennis is a great sport. It brings people together. The story in the book helps to motivate kids to want to learn tennis while also learning some life lessons too. Tennis is a life-time sport. You need minimal equipment and there are many courts available at nearby parks.

In addition to creating this book, we also did a shoe drive in memory of Alan. Our family and friends collected more than 2,174 pairs of shoes that we donated to Soles4Souls.

Soles4Souls collects gently worn shoes to create sustainable jobs and provide relief through the distribution of shoes around the world. The organization has a great mission to wear out poverty. The reason we chose Soles4Souls is because Alan used to always make sure everyone wore a good pair of shoes. In his honor our family will continue to collect and donate shoes.

After you wear out your tennis shoes, please consider giving them to Soles4Souls. Go to their website to find a drop off place near where you live or donate directly at **www.Soles4souls.org**.

Welcome to the "**JUST LOVE TENNIS 4 KIDS**" book.

The word LOVE in the game of tennis means NOTHING or ZERO.

To USPTA Coach Rachelle Lifpitz it means EVERYTHING.

Coach Rachelle just loves teaching kids tennis, and that's why she wrote this book to share with everyone.

What you will find in reading and coloring this book to your kids and grandkids is enjoying the "LOVE" story. You too will feel the LOVE of this great sport called tennis!

Parents, grandparents and coaches can use this as a guide with easy verbal EXPLANATION BOXES to teach the love of tennis.

All you have to know is how to throw a ball underhand.

As you go step by step through the pages of this book you will begin to

"**JUST LOVE TENNIS 4 KIDS**"

This book will not only teach a sport but a sport for a life-time. Kids start around 3 years old and play until they can't play any more. Coach Rachelle is still teaching and watching people in their 80's play!

Tennis keeps the body fit. In an hour of singles play you can burn 580-640 calories. According to a 2016 Harvard University study, playing tennis 3 times a week promotes a longer life.

"In a study done by Johns Hopkins University, tennis strengthens the heart, muscular system and bones."

Playing tennis helps agility, balance, hand–eye coordination and reaction time all while learning sportsmanship skills too.

Another reason to play tennis is to increase your brain power to be more alert, problem solve and relieve stress. "In addition, tennis enhances the neural connections in your brain according to a USTA Study 2013." Kids who play tennis a few times a week tend to do better in school.

Tennis will also aid in developing a positive personality in your children.

Tennis is also great for the whole family to come together and play!

In this book you will find it easier to play tennis by reading and coloring the story first. Then each day go to the court with the book and flow one page at a time, reading only the Explanation Boxes to the kids. This will be easier than you think. Having the correct size racket, smaller courts, nets, and lower-bouncing balls will help aid in learning the game so much faster.

So get started on this life-time sport! "**JUST LOVE TENNIS 4 KIDS**"

Table of Contents

Equipment: Racket Sizes --- 1
Red, Orange, Green Dot, Yellow Balls
Court Sizes for the right age --- 2
Explanation: Pages 1-2 are for the Coach and Parents

Meet Addi! --- 3
Meet Netty! --- 4
Parts of the Racket --- 5
Rules of the Racket --- 6
Table: Names of the Court --- 7
Lines of the court and types of surfaces --- 8
Rules of the Court --- 9
Simon Says Game --- 10

Shake Hands --- 11
Ready Position --- 12
Foot Stance --- 13
Shoulder warm up --- 14
Hand-Eye Coordination --- 15
The Ice Cream Game --- 16
Warm up Feet "Caterpillar Game" --- 17
Pick up the balls…. Make a pizza on the Racket --- 18
Green light, Yellow light, Red light and Purple light --- 19
Volleys: Forehand and Backhand --- 20
Volley foot work (clocks) --- 21
Princess and Prince Game --- 22

Forehand Ground Stroke --- 23
Backhand Ground Stroke --- 24
Hockey Game --- 25
Clean Your Room Game --- 26
Rally --- 27

Lobbing --- 28
Overhead Smash --- 29
Overhead Smash Game --- 30
Serving --- 31

Scoring --- 32
Match Play --- 33
Game Set Match --- 34
A Full Match --- 35
Stretch and Cool Down --- 36
A Full Heart --- 37

Equipment

 ## Coach and Parent Explanation Box:

Parents, Grandparents and Coaches will need to go to their local tennis shop or sporting goods store to purchase a racket, dampener and some red, orange, and green dot balls. A ball hopper or ball tube are also a good piece of equipment to purchase in order to help collect the balls on the court.

A 10' mini portable net for the red court and ball needs to be purchased if the kids are 7 years old and under.

Listed below you will find what size rackets and which color ball your kids should play with, and which size court they should play on. This list is just a guideline. Some kids that are very tall may need to go up in size.

Now locate a tennis court near you. There are many free tennis courts all around the city parks. Tennis is a great way to get the whole family, friends and class mates moving and exercising together!

Enjoy and most of all just have fun!

Racket Size

Ages: 3-4yrs, **Size 19"**
Ages: 5-7yrs **Size 21"or 23"**
Court Size: (36'X18')
Ball Color: **Red**

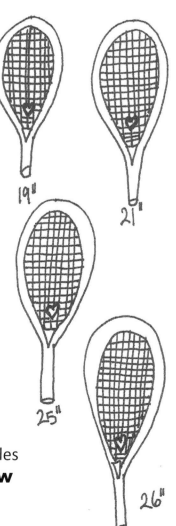

Ages: 8-9yrs **Size 25"**
Court Size: (60'X21' Singles) (60'X27' Doubles)
Ball Color: **Orange**

Ages: 10+yrs **Size 26"**
Full Court Size: (78'X27' Singles) (78'X36') Doubles
Ball Color: **Green Dot** or **standard Yellow**

Court Sizes

Coach and Parent Explanation Box:

The Court size should match the kids age and ability. The appropriate sized racket in hand and slower bouncing balls will all set the kids up for success. A shorter court will help them cover the court for their size.

Having all three makes it easier to learn and they can start to play games. By using this guide below you will know the right size court and ball to use. Help the kids find their right ball and court size.

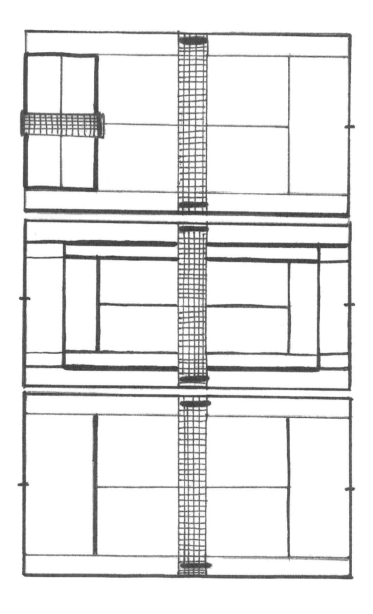

Red Ball and Red Court

Ages: 3-4yrs 5-7yrs
Size Court: 36'x18'

Orange Ball and Orange Court

Ages: 8-10yrs
Size Court:
60'x21' (Singles)
60'x27' (Doubles)

Green Dot Ball (Full Court)

Yellow Ball (Full Court)

Ages: 10+yrs
Court Size:
78'x27' (Singles)
78'x36' (Doubles)

Meet Addi!

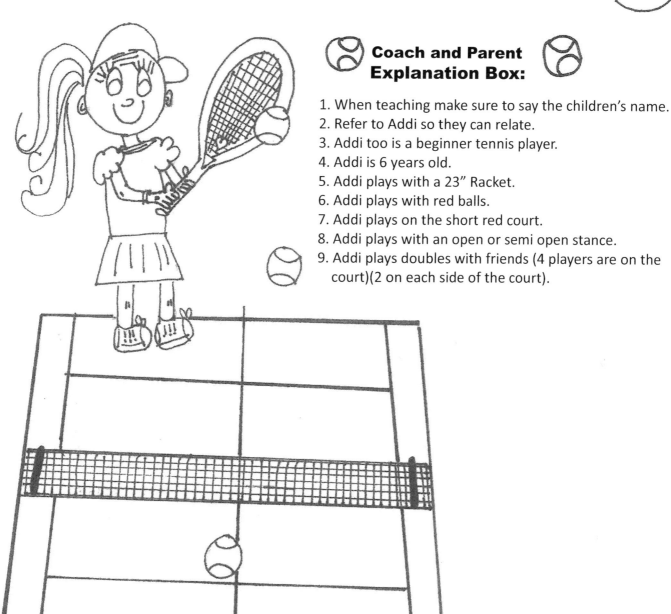

Coach and Parent Explanation Box:

1. When teaching make sure to say the children's name.
2. Refer to Addi so they can relate.
3. Addi too is a beginner tennis player.
4. Addi is 6 years old.
5. Addi plays with a 23" Racket.
6. Addi plays with red balls.
7. Addi plays on the short red court.
8. Addi plays with an open or semi open stance.
9. Addi plays doubles with friends (4 players are on the court)(2 on each side of the court).

This is Addi. She is 6 years old. She is learning to play Tennis! She has a 23" racket that she got at the tennis shop with her grandma. She plays with red balls, on a (36'X 18') red short court. Her favorite stroke is backhand ground stroke, with a open or semi open stance.

She plays the AD court when she plays doubles with Netty. Doubles is when there are two people on each side of the court.

Coach and Parent Explanation Box:

Meet Netty!

1. When teaching make sure to say the children's name.
2. Refer to Netty so they can relate.
3. Netty too is a beginner tennis player.
4. Netty is 8 years old.
5. Netty plays with a 25" racket.
6. Netty plays with both red and orange balls.
7. Netty plays on the red and orange court.
8. Netty plays with a square, open or a semi open stance.

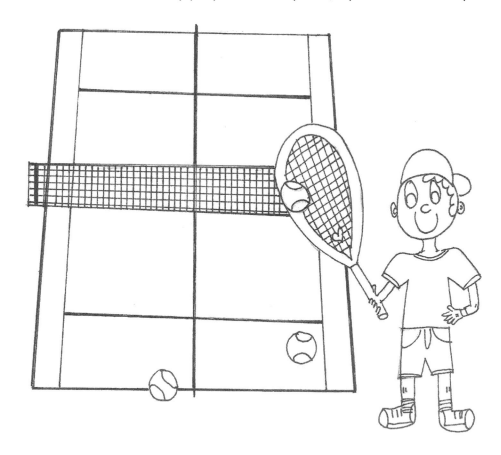

This is Netty. He is 8 years old. He is also learning to play Tennis! He loves his forehand ground stroke. He has a 25" racket. He's been playing for a while so this is his second racket his dad bought for him. He plays with both red and orange balls, mostly orange, unless he plays with Addi, then he uses the red balls only.

They also use the smallest court (36'X18') Netty will play the Deuce side when playing doubles with Addi. When he plays with his 8-10 years age group, he uses the orange balls and the bigger court (60'X27') for doubles. He really likes singles a lot too. When he plays singles, he uses square, open and semi open stance with the orange ball and (60'X21') court size for singles. Singles is when there is only one person on each side of the court.

Coach and Parent Explanation Box:

1. Help the kids name the parts of the racket:
head, face, neck, handle, butt, dampener, frame

PARTS OF THE RACKET

Table:
1. Head
2. Face (Strings)
3. Neck
4. Handle
5. Butt
6. Dampener (Stops vibration)
7. Frame

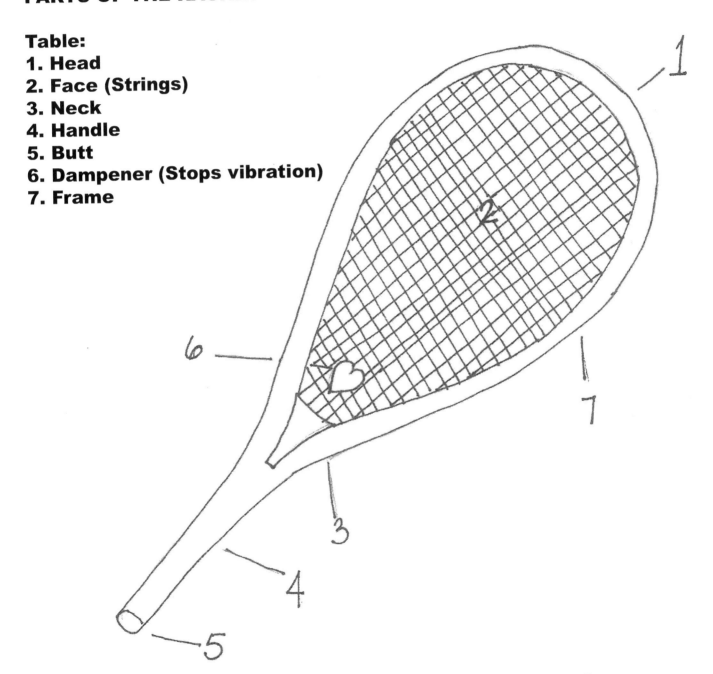

Addi and Netty name the parts of the racket. Addi goes first she says, "Face." Netty goes next he says, "Butt" then they both laugh!

RULES OF THE RACKET

 Coach and Parent Explanation Box:

1. Safety First!
2. Hug the racket like a Bear.
3. Place racket in a racket case when not in use.
4. Only swing the racket at a ball.

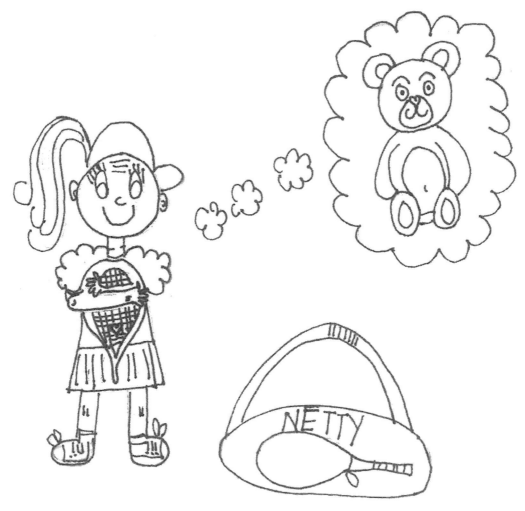

Addi and Netty are learning the rules of the racket. They hug their racket like a bear, when they are not playing with it. They hold their rackets close to make sure they don't accidently hurt someone. Netty likes to put his racket away in a racket case when he's done playing for the day.

Names of The Court

 Coach and Parent Explanation Box:

1. Teach the kids the names of the court.
2. Teach the kids the different court surfaces.
3. Teach the kids the 4 Grand Slam Tournaments.

NAMES OF THE COURT :

1. Net
2. Net Post
3. "T" (in the center of the Service Line)
4. Service Line
5. Deuce Service Box
6. Ad Service Box
7. Singles Line
8. Doubles Line (Alley)
9. Baseline
10. Singles Server (where to stand)
11. Double Server (where to stand)

There are 3 different court surfaces: These surfaces are used in all the 4 Grand Slams, they are the biggest Professional tournaments. The 4 are The Australian Open (Hard Court), The French Open (Clay), Wimbledon (Grass), and US Open (Hard Court).

12. Clay
13. Grass
14. Hard

Lines of the Court and Surfaces

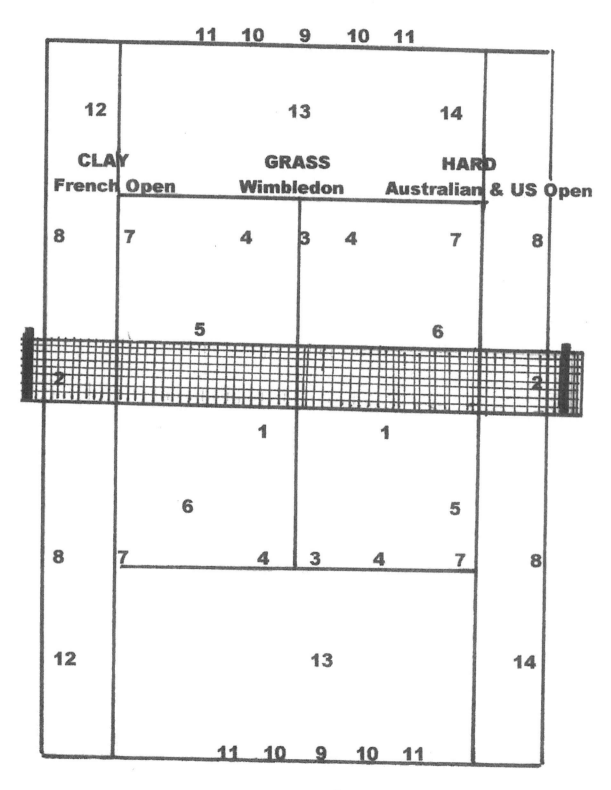

RULES OF THE COURT

 Coach and Parent Explanation Box:

1. Read the rules to the kids before starting to play.
2. Keep this handy to refer to.

1. Always use good sportsmanship
2. Make sure to shake hands when you meet your opponent and when you are finished
3. Tennis is a game of truth
4. Call the shots as you see them IN OR OUT.
5. When the ball touches a line it's IN!
6. Net...Never touch the net with your racket or body (the result is you lose the point)
7. Never reach over the net with your racket or body (the result is you lose the point)
8. Server gets 2 serves unless the ball touches the net. If the ball touches the net on the serve what happens?
   First Serve: It's called a "LET"(only if it lands in the box you get 2 more serves.
   If it does not land in the box, you get one more serve.
   Second Serve: It's called a let you get one more serve, only if it went in the box.
9. The server needs to make sure to always call the score out loud so everyone can hear it. If the returner does not touch the ball and it's in, this is called an ACE. The server ACED his opponent!
10. No talking unless the ball is on your side. If you or your partner talk when the balls is on your opponent's side, it can result in a point for your opponents.
11. When do you change ends of the court?
    Then change ends of the court on odd number of games played.
    Example: 4 to 1=5 this is odd
12. Once you have explained the rules remember the most important one is to just have fun!

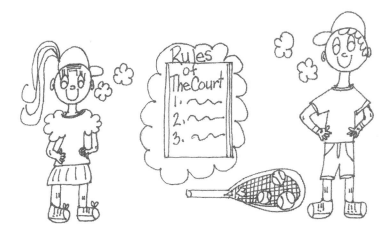

Addi and Netty are reading the rules of the court sheet with their parents because they aren't sure of a rule. Addi called a ball out that landed on her side. Netty thought his ball was in. They did not know who got the point.

So they asked their parents and they didn't know either. They decided to read the rules of the court sheet. The answer was in the rules of the court. Addi was right. The ball is hers to call in or out, when on her side of the court. So the ball was out and Addi received the point. Netty understood and showed great sportsmanship.

Simon Says Game

  Coach and Parent Explanation Box:

1 Call out Simon Says, then name a line or part of the court. Use the Line names from Table on page 7
2. Kids run to the line or part of the court! Only if Simon says!
3. If Simon does not say and they run to it, then they are out..
4. Cheer on the others, like a good sportsman.
5. Last child standing is the winner! Learning the lines of the court will help stimulate their brains.
6. Who would have thought having so much fun could help kids get better grades too!

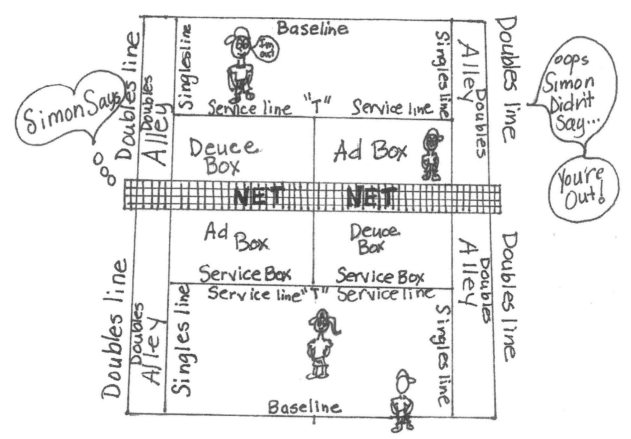

Addi and Netty learn the lines of the court by playing a game called Simon Says.

They like to play it with their friends. It helps them remember the lines and parts of the court, like the net (for Netty) and Ad court (for Addi). They can't forget those names! Netty's friend wanted to play too, but he did not know how to play. Netty said." I will teach him." Netty said this is an Example: If Simon Says, run to the baseline and you run to it, (if your guess is right) you stay and play more, if it's wrong you're out of the game.

If Simon does not say and you go then you are out of the game. "If you want to be a good sport you can cheer us on" said Netty, until last one is standing. The last one standing is the winner! Also, you can get out too by Example: Go to the Net Netty yells and oops his friend run to the net, but Simon did not say. He is out. Again the last one standing is the winner! Now its your turn to play Simon Says, so you too can learn the lines and parts of the Tennis Court!

Shake Hands

 Coach and Parent Explanation Box:

1. Put the racket in the child's dominant hand.
2. Shake hands with the racket.
3. This is called the Continental shake hands grip.

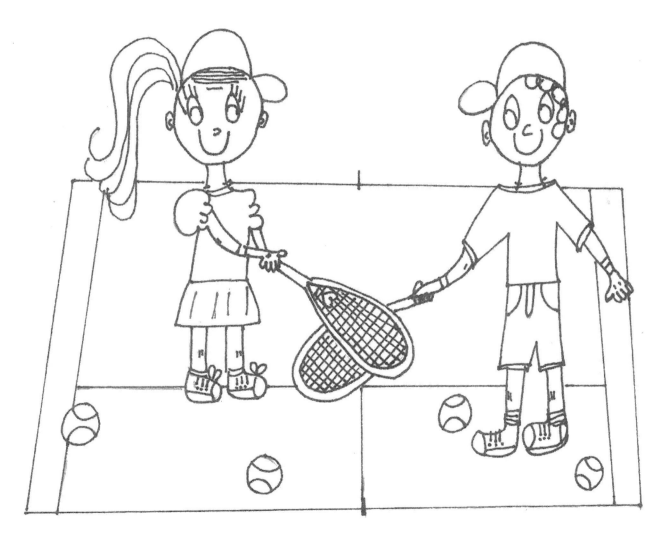

Netty shows Addi how to hold the tennis racket. They both hold the racket with their right hand, (because they write with their right hand.) They hold the racket all the way down by the Butt of the racket. Now they are laughing and having fun shaking hands with their rackets. Now it's your turn to hold the racket and shake hands with it!

Ready Position

 Coach and Parent Explanation Box:

1. Hold the racket with two hands
   (dominant hand is on the handle other hand is on the neck).
2. Bounce on their toes.
3. Bent Knees.
4. Pretend the racket is a pencil.

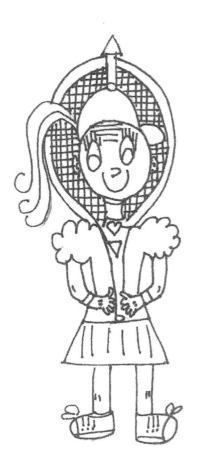 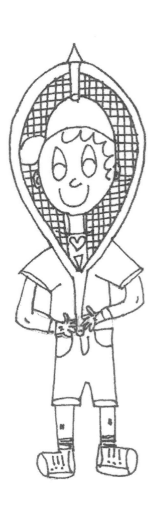

Addi and Netty get into Ready Position, holding the racket with two hands, (dominant hand is on the handle, other hand is on the neck). They are bouncing on their toes, leaning forward with their knees bent. The racket position is forward. They like to pretend their racket is a pencil (the point is on the top of the racket head) because they love to draw hearts.

Foot Stance

Coach and Parent Explanation Box:

1. Ready Position!
2. Pre Rally kids 3-5 years old
   open and semi stance (forehand and back hand).
3. Rallying Kids 5-10 years old
   square, semi open and open stance (forehand or backhand).
4. Square and semi stance during a rally, open stance on wide and fastballs.

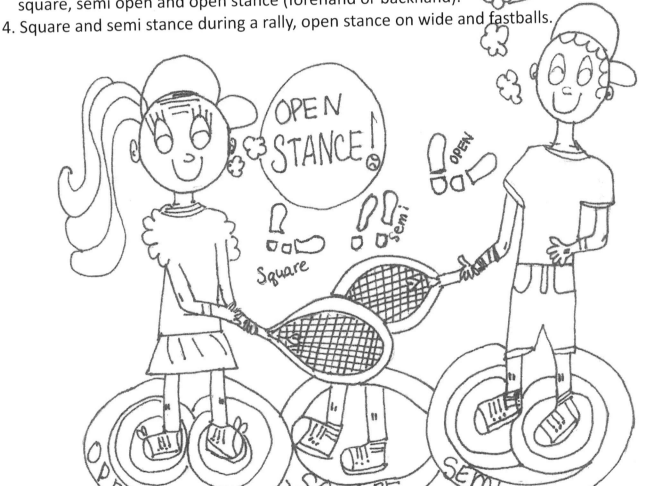

Addi and Netty get into ready position. They show each other the different foot stances they use. They both started tennis when they were 3 years old using red balls on the red court. They used open and semi stance then.

They still use open and semi stance. Now that Netty is more advanced moving to the orange court and orange balls he uses square, open and semi stance too.

When he rallies (hitting the ball back and forth) he uses the square and semi stance. He uses open stance for wide and fastballs too.

Shoulder Warm Up

 Coach and Parent Explanation Box:

1. Pretend the racket is a pencil and at the head of the racket is the point (Engaging the MIND).
2. Draw hearts on both right and left sides of the body.
3. Follow the arrows.
4. This warms up the shoulders (Engaging the BODY).
5. This warm up draws a full heart (Engaging the SOUL).

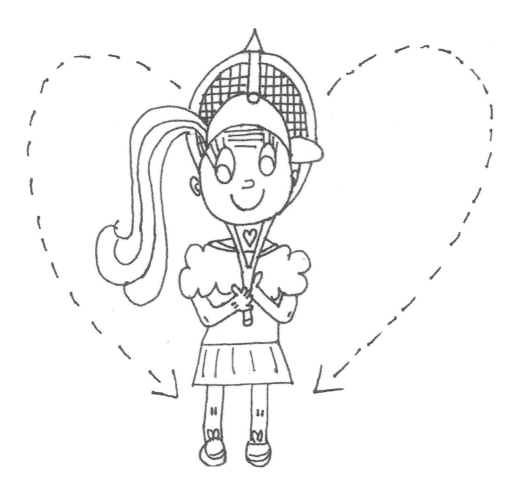

Addi is demonstrating how to warm up her shoulders by imagining the racket is a pencil (at the head of the racket is the point). She likes to think about drawing a heart. Addi draws one side of the heart (forehand) and then other side of the heart, (backhand) following the arrows. As you can see it makes a full heart.

Addi can feel herself making hearts as she warms her shoulders. She expresses the love of tennis by making a full heart. This makes Addi's Mind, Body and Soul feel so happy! She just loves tennis!

Hand-Eye Coordination

 Coach and Parent Explanation Box:

Hand –Eye Coordination
Doing this drill with your kids can help improve their agility, balance, coordination, and reaction time. This skill game will contribute to good hand-eye coordination.
Starting hand-eye coordination at such a young age helps them with many other activities.
The best way to form muscle memory is to start at a young age. Have the kids count and see how many they can do in the row.

1. With a ball and racket bounce the ball down by pushing the ball down or up.
2. Have the kids count how many they can do in 1 minute.
3. Have them remember their record and try to beat it the next time.

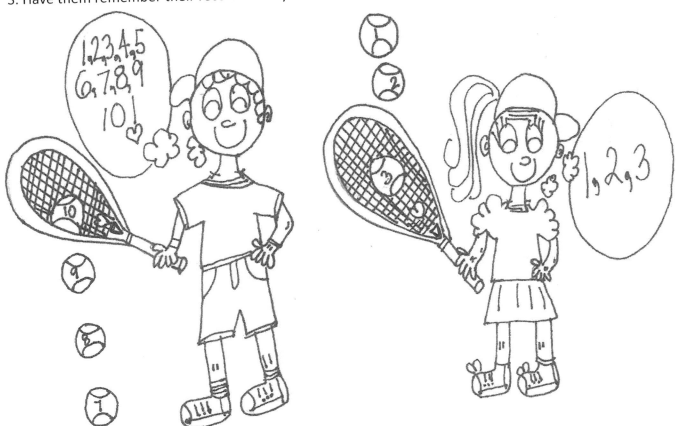

Watch Addi and Netty hit balls down on the racket. That's when the ball hits their racket and they hit down on the ball. They try to do this as many times in a row as they can, without missing. They also do ups. That's when you put the ball on your racket and you push up, letting the ball come down and hit your racket without missing.

Addi can bounce the ball down eight times and up three times. Netty's record is ten down and five up. Now let's see how many you can get in a row!

The Ice Cream Game

Coach and Parent Explanation Box:

1. Even number of kids line up across from each other in the alley.
2. One child has the three balls and the other one has a cone with the cone upside down, so the hole is facing up.
3. The child with the three balls throws a ball one at a time into the cone, while calling out their favorite ice cream.
4. The kids switch position so the other person can make an ice cream cone too!
5. The object is to get all three balls in the cone! This is called a Triple Decker ice cream cone!

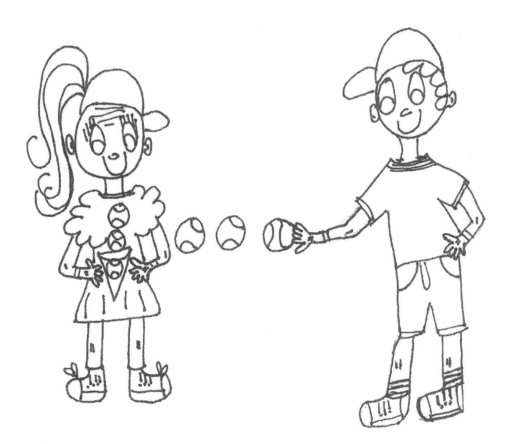

Addi and Netty love the ice cream game. They pretend the balls are their favorite flavors of ice cream. Let's learn to play the ice cream game, this too helps with hand-eye coordination. Addi holds the cone and Netty throws one ball at a time into the cone, calling out his favorite flavors.

Netty made a triple decker of chocolate, cookie dough and mint chip. They take turns holding the cone and throwing. Now it's your turn to make your favorite ice cream cone.

Coach and Parent Explanation Box:

1. Line up in one line at the "T".
2. Parent coach throws (under hand).
3. Red Ball side to side back and forth.
4. Kids split-step (spread legs apart)).
5. Trying to get the ball between their legs.
6. If the kids miss the ball they get an X.
7. When they have 3 X'S you are out.
8. Last one with the least X's wins.

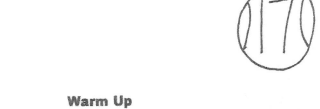
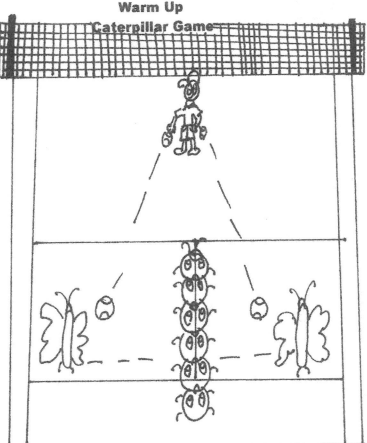

Addi and Netty's favorite warm up game is called Caterpillar. It gets their whole body moving, especially their arms and feet.

Addi and Netty run to the "T" and line up in a straight line with their friends. They all pretend they are first caterpillars, as they move their arms they will feel more like butterflies. Addi's mom throws the ball low to the ground, from side to side moving everyone. Addi and Netty and their friends stay together as if they are a caterpillar moving together. They run to the ball and split their legs apart to let the ball go threw their legs. They all flap their arms like they are flying.

The faster they move the more beautiful the butterflies fly.

Netty shuffles with Addi and his friends then split-steps (spreads legs apart) to get the ball through his legs but hits his leg now Netty needs to go to the back of the line and he gets a X. He is a good sport and knows it's OK because he has two more X's. When someone get 3 X's they are out. Addi is so happy because she shuffles with her friends then spit steps (spreads legs apart) and the ball goes through. She gets to continue the game.They play this game a few more times and most of the kids are getting , X's !Addi is the last one standing with only one X . She's so happy! She is the winner! Addi feels like a beautiful butterfly.

Pick up Ball
Make a Pizza on the Racket

 Coach and Parent **Explanation Box:**

1. Put all rackets on the ground.
2. Have the kids collect the balls as fast as they can.
3. Put the balls on the racket.
4. Time them to see how fast they can make a pizza on their racket.
5. Then have them put the pizza in the oven (cart).

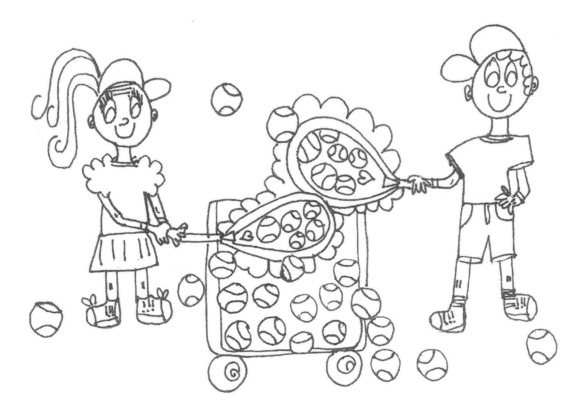

The easiest way to collect balls is to collect them on your racket to put them back in the cart. Addi and Netty like to pretend to make a pizza on their racket. First they collect balls for the first layer calling it crust. The next layer of balls will be the sauce. Then you add the cheese last comes the toppings. Add anything you would like to the pizza. Addi loves to put gummy bears on top of her pizza. Netty likes cherries. Now that we have complete pizzas, it is time to put them in the oven. We use the ball cart as the oven. It is so much fun for Addi and Netty they

JUST LOVE PIZZA! Now it's your turn to see if you can balance the balls on the racket and put the pizza in the oven.

Green light, Yellow light, Red light and Purple light

 Coach and Parent Explanation Box:

A. Kids move about the court by:
  1. Shuffling
  2. Running
  3. Skipping
  4. Jumping

B. Call out :
  1. Green Light = GO
  2. Yellow Light = SLOW
  3. Red Light = STOP
  4. Purple Light = DANCE

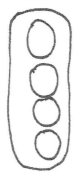
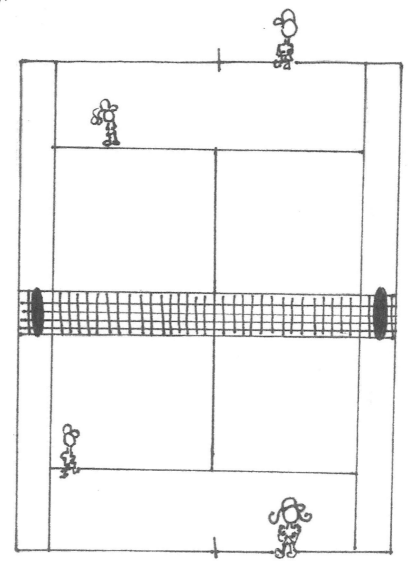

Another warm up game to get the body moving is Green light, Yellow light, Red light and Purple light! They start by listening to their Coach or Parent call out a color. Green light was called, so everyone was running or skipping super fast. Then Yellow light was called, so we all slowed down shuffling side to side slowly. Next Red light was called, everyone STOPPED!

After a few minutes Purple light was called! Everyone loves Purple light because you get to DANCE! We all like to show off our dance moves.

Volley's Forehand and Backhand

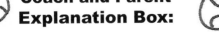
**How to hit a forehand and backhand volley
Coach and Parent
Explanation Box:**

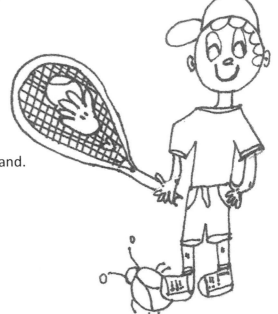

1. Kids need to be in ready position.
2. Forehand: racket in right or (lefty left hand) dominant.
3. Forehand: racket face is on the right side (Left side for lefty).
4. Backhand: 2 hands on the racket on the left side (for a righty) Right side for lefty.
5. Backhand: Dominant hand always goes first, then the other hand.
6. Parent Coach tosses (under hand) to the racket.

Netty is demonstrating how to hit a forehand volley. He starts with his racket in ready position. We learned this in a previous page. He turns his left shoulder to the right. Netty turns to the right because he is right handed. Please note, if someone is left handed, they would turn to the left. While doing so, he transfers the racket into his right hand. Now he is ready to work on his footwork. Netty steps his left foot forward, calling out ,"step on the bug"! The last step is making contact with the ball. Netty likes to scream out high five as he is hitting the ball over the net. Step on the bug, and high five the ball.

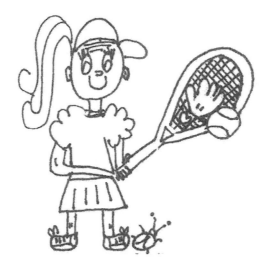

Addi is demonstrating a backhand volley. Her racket is in ready position. This time she keeps two hands on the racket and turns her shoulders to the left. Addi is also right handed. Remember if someone is left handed, they will turn their shoulder to the left. Now it's time to step on the bug and high five the ball. Addi steps forward with her right foot. Our left-handed players will step forward with their left foot. Remember backhands require two hands.

Volley (footwork) Clocks

 Coach and Parent Explanation Box:

1. Match the numbers on both clocks, for Forehand or Backhand.
2. Volley Clocks: tell kids to place racket and feet @12,o'clock,1,3 or 12,11,9.
3. Clocks will help with footwork and Hand-Eye coordination.
4. Throw under hand to the racket.

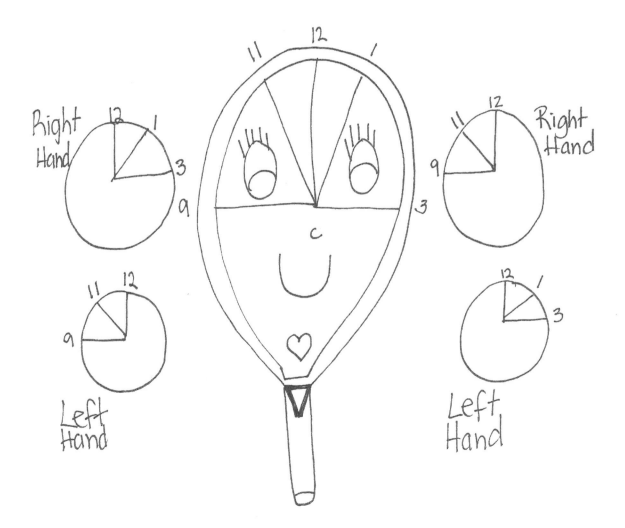

Netty and Addi love to volley back and forth over the net! Addi loves to pretend she's stepping on a bug and high five-ing the ball. She giggles every time. The clocks really help Addi and Netty. It helps them remember where to place the racket and where to step on the bug. Now you try thinking about the clock. Does it help you?

Princess and Prince Game

Coach and Parent Explanation Box:

1. Kids line up at the net.
2. Coach or Parent throws a ball under hand towards the racket. (forehand) and (Backhand).
3. Kids volley the ball over the net they continue 1,2,3,4,5, Forehand then after all 5 then (Backhand).
4. If the ball does not go over, the net kids will go to the (Alley)
5. If the kids can get the ball over five times in a row, then they become a Princess or a Prince

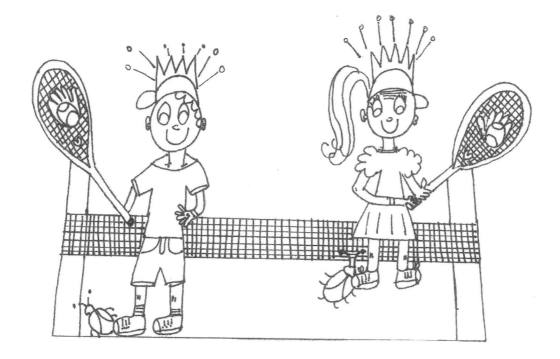

Addi and Netty love to play the volley game with their friends. Now it is time to learn the game too with Addi and Netty.
The Princess and Prince game is so much fun.

Addi and Netty and their friends line up against the net. All the kids have their rackets in ready position. Netty's Grandpa Joe throws (under hand) a ball over the net towards their racket, and the kids hit it. They remember, step on the bug and high five the ball.
If the ball goes over the net then everyone stays and continue to hit balls until five volleys in a row.

If they miss a ball, they go into the alley. They stay there until the next person gets all the balls over and free them. When Addi, Netty and all their friends get five balls over in a row, they become a princess or a prince. Then they all high five each other and say, "Good Job!"

Forehand Ground Stroke

 Coach and Parent Explanation Box:

1. Start in ready position.
2. Pretend the racket is a pencil.
3. Draw one side of the heart (Right) (opposite for lefty).
4. Square stance (Neutral).
5. Meet the ball in front.
6. Once the ball is hit, then finish with a big bag of toys over the (left) shoulder (opposite for lefty).
7. Catches the racket over his shoulder with both hands.
7. Make sure to bring the back leg around to meet the front leg.
8. Back to Ready Position.

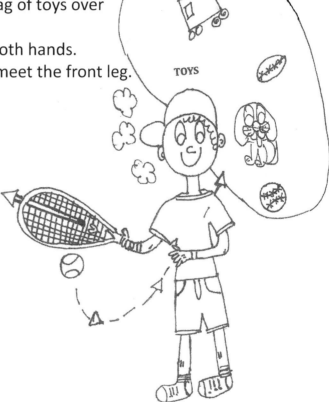

Netty loves to hit forehand ground strokes.

When he plays doubles with Addi he plays the deuce side because he loves his forehand so much. He knows how to hit a forehand groundstroke every well.

He starts in ready position, square stance. He likes to pretend his racket is a pencil. He turns his left shoulder to the right then he pictures himself drawing the right side of a heart. He meets the ball in front, then swings it over his (left) shoulder, like he's throwing a large bag of toys over his (left) shoulder, and catching the racket with both hands. He needs to make sure he is ready for his next ball so he brings his back foot (right) around to meet the other foot. Now Netty is back in ready position and ready for the next ball!

Backhand Ground Strokes

 Coach and Parent Explanation Box:

1. Start in ready position.
2. Pretend the racket is a pencil.
3. Draw one side of a heart (Left) side (Opposite for Lefty).
4. Semi Stance.
5. Meet the ball in front.
6. Once the ball is hit then it's time to finish with a big bag of toys over the (Right) shoulder (Opposite for Lefty).
7. Make sure to bring the back leg around to meet the front leg.
8. Back to ready Position.

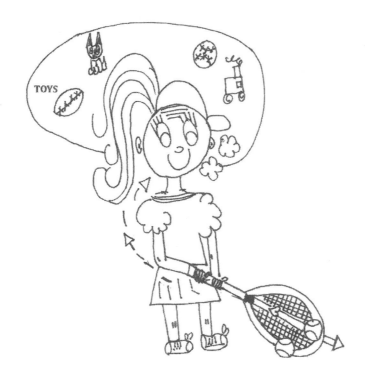

Addi's favorite stroke is the backhand ground stroke. Watch how she hits the ball. She starts in ready position. Then keeping both hands on the racket, she turns her right shoulder. She also likes to pretend her racket is a pencil. She draws the left side of a heart as she takes her racket back. Then she lunges with her right leg (semi stance), meets the ball then she finishes.

Addi likes to pretend she is throwing a big bag of toys over her (right) shoulder when she finishes the stroke. Also, she brings her (left) leg around to meet the front leg. Now she is back to ready position to hit the next ball. Now it's your turn to try hitting a backhand this way!

Hockey Game

 Coach and Parent Explanation Box:

1. Set up cones on both sides.
2. Space cones far enough apart so the kids can make a goal.
3. The object is to get ten goals (the ball through the cones).
4. Block the ball from not going through the cones is good eye-hand coordination.

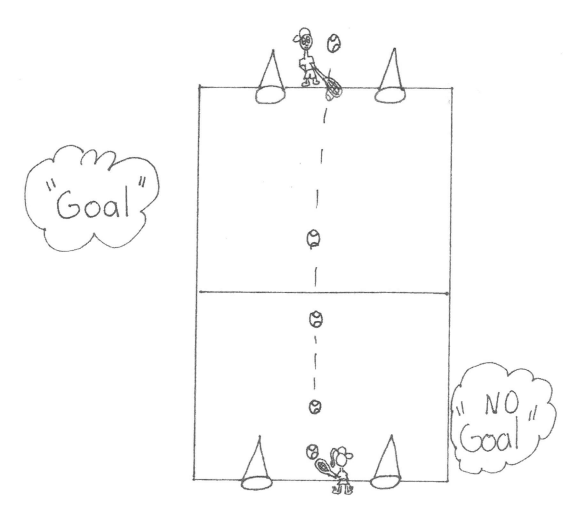

Addi and Netty enjoy playing, Hockey with one another. It's a very challenging game. The most fun is when the ball goes in between the cones and someone scores a goal. The first one to get 10 goals is the winner!

Clean Your Room Game

Coach and Parent Explanation Box:

1. Put twenty balls on each side of the court.
2. Same number of kids on each side.
3. Cheer them on to see which side is clean first.
4. Who's ever room is cleaned first is the winner.

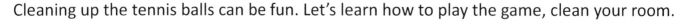

NETTY'S ROOM IS CLEAN!!!!

Cleaning up the tennis balls can be fun. Let's learn how to play the game, clean your room.

Addi and her friends are on one side of the court and Netty and his friends are on the other side.

The kids put twenty balls on each side of the court. Now they are ready to play the game. Each side at the same time, bounces the ball and hits a groundstroke over to the opposite side of the court. The team with no balls left wins!

Let's see if you can clean your room as fast as Netty and his friends!

Rally

 Coach and Parent Explanation Box:

1. One or two players on one side of the court and others on the other side.
2. Bounce the ball and hit it over the net.
3. Kids need to count how many times they can hit the ball over the net.

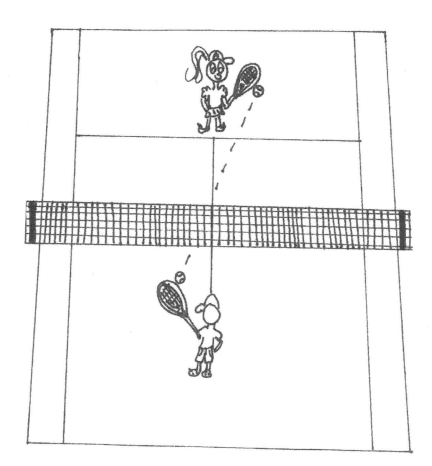

Addi hits the tennis ball over the net then Netty hits the ball over the net.

This is called a rally or rallying. Addi loves to hit back and forth. She tells Netty to count how many they can hit in a row without missing. Sometimes they can get up to five hits in a row. Let's see how many you can hit in a row.

Lobbing

 Coach and Parent Explanation Box:

1. Kids need to drop their pencil (racket head).
2. Sweep the floor and shoot the ball up to the sky over their shoulder.

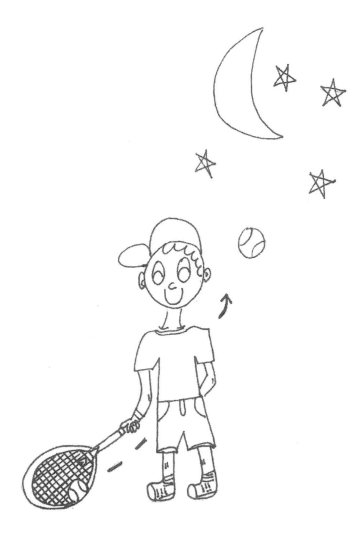

Netty is learning to lob. Lobs can be done on the forehand and backhand side. A lob is when a ball goes very high, and deep to the baseline. When people are at the net lobbing over their head is a good way to win a point.

Netty shows how to lob, by dropping the head of the racket, then sweeping the floor then, driving the ball straight up to the stars in the sky. Teaching the kids to drop the racket like Netty will help them have a great lob.

Overhead Smash

 Coach and Parent Explanation Box:

1. Put the racket over shoulder.
2. Reach up to the sky and point index figure at the ball.
3. Meet the ball then smash it.
4. Finish by the other side of your ankle.

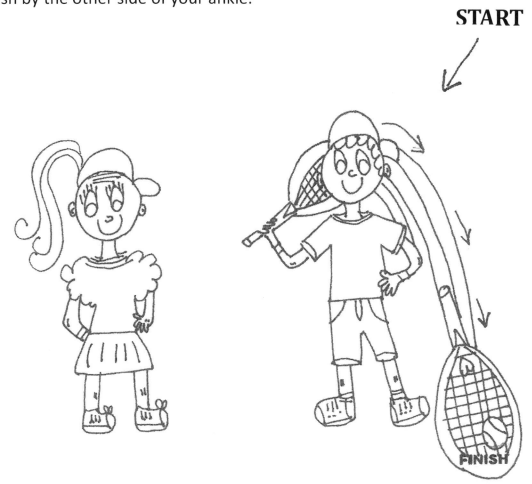

Netty shows Addi how to hit an overhead smash.

Netty says,"Just turns sideways towards the net post, on an angle at 1:00 on the clock." He points at the ball like this (with his index finger,) leaning back with all his weight on his heels. Then he puts the racket over his shoulder just behind his head like this!

Netty says to Addi,"When you see the ball high in the air, that's when you want to shift your weight forward to the ball." He reaches high in the sky to show her. Then he smashes it and finishing with the racket at the other side of his ankle. "Overhead smashes are so much fun!", said Addi.

Overhead Smash Game

 Coach and Parent Explanation Box:

1. Have kids lob three times.
2. After three lobs they play the point out.(with whatever stroke).
3. First one to win ten points is a winner!

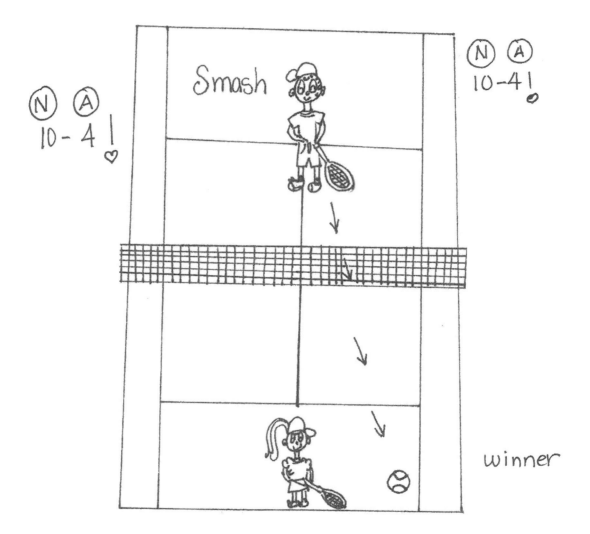

Addi and Netty play the lobbing game together. Addi lobs to Netty then Netty lobs back. They lob three times then Netty does a overhead smash and wins the point. The first one to 10 is the winner. The score was 10-4 Netty won! Addi says,"You're strong!" Netty says, "Do you want to feel my muscle?"

Serving

 Coach and Parent Explanation Box:

1. Face the net post and point the left foot towards the net post (for right handed players) (opposite for left handed players) right foot points at the net post.
2. Racket goes over their shoulder.
3. Toss the ball up to the sky.
4. Smash it. (Like a overhead smash).
5. Tell kids to pretend they are going over the rainbow to the pot of gold!

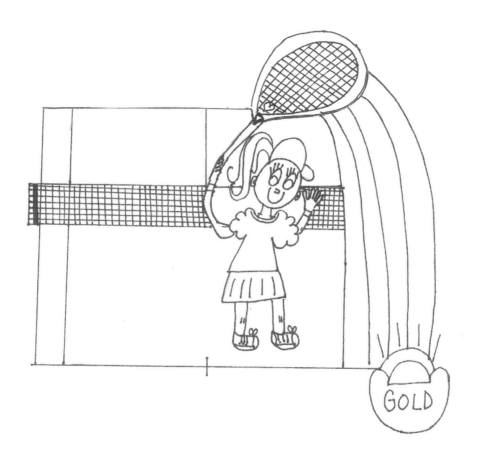

Serving is one of Addi's best strokes. Having a good serve is important, because it's the first stroke of the game. Without it you can't start the game.

Addi starts by turning her body towards the right net post with her left foot pointing at the net post too. Then she pretends the ball is a baby bird in a nest in her hand. She then releases the ball up to the sky. Addi has her racket over her shoulder, then when the ball is at it's peak Addi reaches for the stars, and tries to smash the ball on her racket (like a overhead smash). Addi likes to think she is going over a rainbow to the pot of gold. The pot of gold is by her left ankle, where she finishes her stroke.

Scoring

 Coach and Parent Explanation Box:

1. Learn to score a tennis game, tiebreaker, set, and a whole match.
2. Ages: 3-4 year old just to count 1,2,3,4, point they win a game! They can play as many games as they want.
3. Ages: 5-7 year old play a match one SET first one to 6 games wins! (by 2 games) use regular scoring (with NO AD scoring) This is when after deuce the next point wins!
4. Ages: 8- 10 year old play a match best out of 3 sets first one to 6 games (by 2 games) (NO AD scoring) .

A Scoring:
   1. 0-0 Starts the first match score Then say the game score Love –Love(Love means "0")
   2. 1st point 15
   3. 2nd point 30
   4. 3rd point 40
   5. 4th point Game

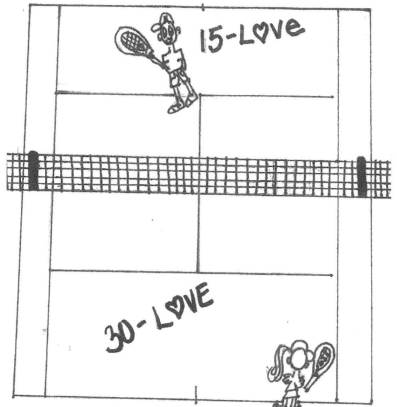

Addi and Netty play a few games to practice keeping score.

The person that is serving is the one calling out the score. They always call their score first. Netty is starting on the deuce side to start the game. He calls the score out loud so Addi can hear him. He calls out the over all set game score 0-0 and the current games score, Love-Love. He needs to call out the match game score at the start of each game, this is good sportsmanship to call the score loud so all can hear him. Netty wins the next point. He calls the score 15-Love. Netty wins the next point. He calls the score 30-Love. Addi wins the next point so it is now 30-15. Netty wins the next point 40-15. Netty comes in for a point winning volley. He wins this game! Addi says, "Nice game!"

Match Play

 Coach and Parent Explanation Box:

1. **Match Play for ages: 5-7 years old.**
2. Play the first one to six games (win by two) NO AD scoring.
3. Switch sides of the court on odd numbered games.

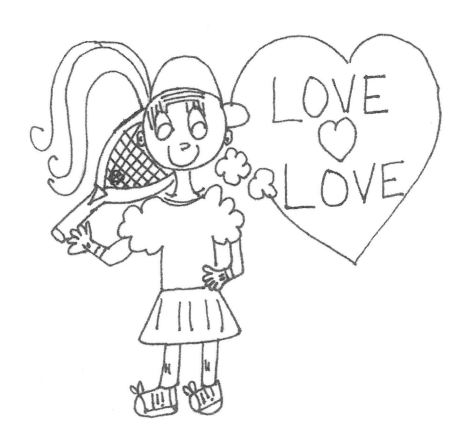

Now it's Addi's turn to serve. So, they switch sides of the court. They remember to switch sides always on odd numbers 1,3,5.... Then Addi starts to serve on the deuce side, by calling out the match score, 0-1 and LOVE-LOVE

Netty wins the next point so the score now is Love-15

Addi wins and the score is 15-15.

Netty wins and the score is 15-30.

Addi wins and the score is 30-30 or 30 all.

Next Addi wins again the score is 40-30.

Netty wins and the score is 40-40 or it is also called deuce.

The next point wins, because there is NO AD scoring.

Netty wins the next point. Netty wins the game!

Game Set Match

 Coach and Parent Explanation Box:

1. First one to six games (within two games) wins.
2. This is called a SET.
3. In a set if you get to 6-6 then a tiebreaker is needed. The first one to get to 7 points by 2 wins.
4. When the match is over, make sure to say, "Nice match!"

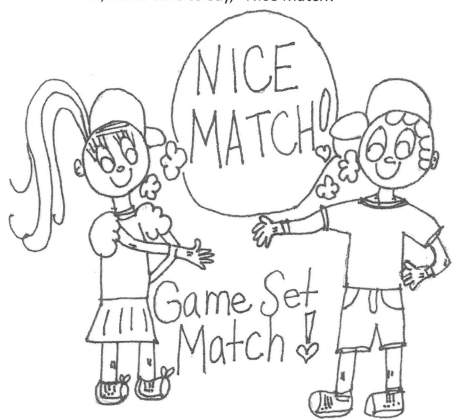

They continue to play! Netty stays on his side of the court (even number) and calls the score. He remembers to call out the match game score at the start of the game. He calls it, 2-0, Love-Love. Addi and Netty continue their match until they get to 6 games (win by two) this is called a Set.

If they get to 6-5 then they play the best of 7 (win by 2).

If they get to 6-6 games then a tiebreaker will be played. This is the first one to 7 points (by 2) wins. Addi and Netty do not need to do a tiebreaker. Netty wins 6-4 games and says "GAME SET MATCH!" They both show great sportsmanship by going to the net and saying, "Nice match!"

A Full Match

 Coach and Parent Explanation Box:

1. Ages: 8-10 years old play best of 3 sets (NO Ad scoring).
2. The goal is to win in 2 sets.
3. If one person wins one set and the other person wins the other...you have to play a tiebreaker.
4. A 10 point tie-breaker (win by 2) will determine who wins!
5. Always be a good sport and say, "Nice Match" at the end.

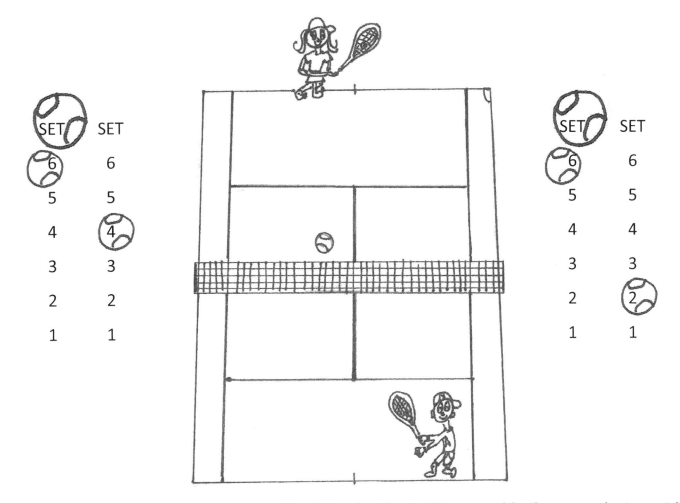

Netty plays a full match with one of his friends. She is 10 years old. They are playing with the green dot ball on a full court. They play the best out of 3 sets (with NO Ad scoring) Netty hopes to win two sets in a row. This way he won't have to go to a tiebreaker (10 points within two) to decide the winner. Netty won in two sets 6-4 6-2! He says, "Game, Set, Match! He then shakes his opponent's hand.

Stretch and Cool Down

 Coach and Parent Explanation Box:

1. When the body is still warm it's a good time to stretch the muscles.
2. As the body cools down you can keep stretching.
3. Talk about the match you just had.
4. Make sure to remind players to be good sports and hosts.
5. Offer a drink and a snack at the end of the match.

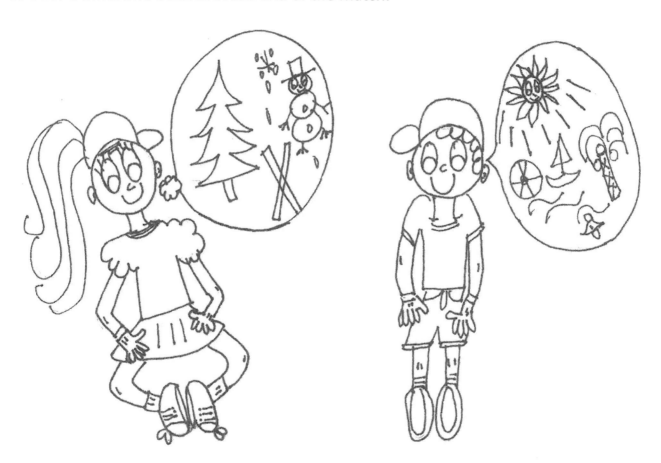

After a long match all players need to drink plenty of water and cool down too.

Addi and Netty sit down on the ground in a circle. Their Coach or Parent says

"Lets stretch." They put their feet together (like airplane wings). The Coach or Parent says," Let pretend we are flying somewhere. Netty said, I'm going to fly to

Los Cabo, Mexico, to go to the beach and surf. Addi wants to fly to Colorado to ski. They also stretch their arms forward towards their feet. This is a good time to talk about how your match went. Now all players have worked up a appetite. It's time to offer everyone a drink and a snack.

A Full Heart

Coach and Parent Explanation Box:

1. Just have fun!

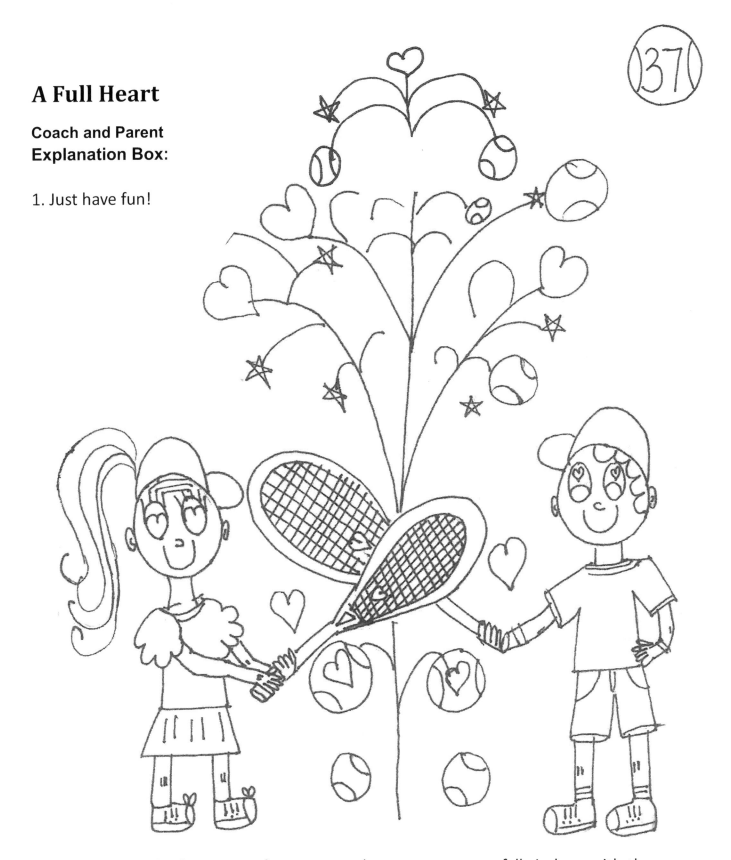

Tennis is called the love game for a reason, because everyone falls in love with the game. Addi and Netty JUST LOVE TENNIS!

They love to inspire and motivate their friends too. They are so excited for the future they have in tennis. Now it's your turn for your future in tennis!

About The Author

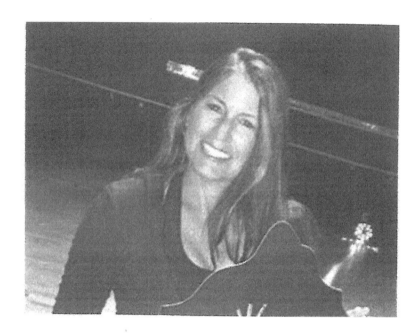

The writer and illustrator, **Rachelle Lifpitz**, is a USPTA (United States Professional Tennis Asso.) Tennis Coach. She has 18 years experience teaching young kids.
She has brought the love of tennis to all the kids she has taught.

Coach Rachelle taught her daughter Samantha Lifpitz from age 3 years old all the way to Division 1 College Tennis.
Samantha played for University of Northern Colorado. She rated #3 in Colorado, 22 Intermountain, 281 Nationally.

Why should you buy this book?
Coach Rachelle wrote this book so that all parents, grandparents and coaches can learn, step by step to teach kids the love of playing a lifetime sport!
Over the years Coach Rachelle has seen kids thrive physically and mentally by moving their bodies playing the game of tennis. Tennis balances the brain.
Coach Rachelle believes playing tennis will help your kids become better students, improve social skills and learn to solve problems all while getting fit.

She also believes tennis helps strengthen the Mind, Body, and Soul of a person.
This book you will not only give the gift of learning a lifetime sport but help in, wearing out poverty, by donating your gently used tennis shoes to Souls4Soles.

"JUST LOVE TENNIS BOOK 4 KIDS" will donate to:
Souls4Soles @ www.Souls4Soles.org

Made in the USA
Middletown, DE
27 September 2023

39496464R00027